BORON CURE
FOR
SENIORS WITH ARTHRITIS

Unlocking Potential for Joint Relief with Boron-

Rich Recipes for Active Aging

JANE THORNTHWAITE

Table of Contents

Chapter 1

Introduction

Types of Arthritis: A Comprehensive Overview

Arthritis encompasses a diverse group of inflammatory joint diseases, each presenting unique symptoms and challenges. The two primary types are osteoarthritis (OA) and rheumatoid arthritis (RA). Osteoarthritis, often associated with aging and wear-and-tear, involves the gradual breakdown of joint cartilage, leading to pain and stiffness. Rheumatoid arthritis, on the other hand, is an autoimmune disorder where the immune system mistakenly attacks joint linings, causing inflammation, pain, and potential deformities.

Other notable forms include gout, characterized by the accumulation of uric acid crystals in joints, and ankylosing spondylitis, primarily affecting the spine. Psoriatic arthritis is linked to the skin condition psoriasis, impacting joints and causing inflammation.

Symptoms across types may include joint pain, swelling, and limited mobility, affecting daily activities. Diagnosis involves a combination of medical history, physical examinations, and imaging tests. While there's no cure for most types of arthritis, management focuses on pain relief, preserving joint function, and improving quality of life. Treatments range from medications to lifestyle modifications, including exercise and weight management.

Understanding the specific type of arthritis is crucial for tailoring effective interventions. A multidisciplinary approach involving rheumatologists, physical therapists, and lifestyle adjustments is often key to mitigating the impact of arthritis on an individual's well-being. Regular monitoring and adapting treatment plans as needed contribute to improved outcomes for those living with arthritis.

The Arthritis Epidemic: Statistics and Impact

The arthritis epidemic poses a significant public health challenge globally. According to recent statistics, over 54 million adults in the United States alone grapple with arthritis, making it a leading cause of disability. The prevalence is expected to rise, with projections estimating that, by 2040, over 78 million Americans will be affected.

Arthritis's impact extends beyond physical discomfort, affecting mental health and overall quality of life. It is a major contributor to work limitations and absenteeism, with billions of dollars spent annually on medical costs and lost earnings. Moreover, the condition disproportionately affects the aging population, adding strain to healthcare systems worldwide.

Efforts to address this epidemic involve public health campaigns promoting arthritis awareness, early detection, and lifestyle interventions to manage symptoms. As the prevalence of arthritis continues to climb, there is a growing imperative for collaborative efforts among healthcare professionals, policymakers, and communities to implement effective strategies for prevention, management, and improved overall well-being for those affected.

Current Treatments for Arthritis

Current treatments for arthritis aim to alleviate pain, reduce inflammation, and improve joint function. Nonsteroidal anti-inflammatory drugs (NSAIDs) like ibuprofen and naproxen are commonly prescribed to manage pain and inflammation. Disease-modifying antirheumatic drugs (DMARDs), such as methotrexate, target the immune system to slow the progression of rheumatoid arthritis.

Biologics, a type of DMARD, are engineered proteins that interfere with specific components of the immune system responsible for inflammation. Corticosteroids may be used to quickly suppress inflammation, particularly in acute cases.

For osteoarthritis, pain management often involves analgesics like acetaminophen or prescription medications. Physical therapy is commonly recommended to improve joint flexibility and strengthen supportive muscles.

Lifestyle modifications, including weight management and regular exercise, play a crucial role in arthritis management. In severe cases, surgical interventions like joint replacement may be considered.

Research continues to explore innovative therapies, including regenerative medicine approaches like stem cell therapy. Personalized treatment plans, often involving a combination of medications and lifestyle adjustments, are tailored to the specific type and severity of arthritis, promoting better outcomes and improved quality of life for individuals living with this condition

The Anatomy of Joints

Joints are vital structures in the human body that facilitate movement and provide flexibility. There are various types of joints, each with its own anatomy and function.

1. **Synovial Joints:**

These are the most common and movable joints. They typically contain a synovial cavity filled with synovial fluid, which lubricates and nourishes the joint. Examples include the knee, hip, and shoulder joints.

2. **Cartilaginous Joints:**

These joints are connected by cartilage, providing slight flexibility. The intervertebral discs in the spine are an example of cartilaginous joints.

3. **Fibrous Joints:**

In fibrous joints, bones are connected by fibrous tissue, offering limited or no movement. Sutures in the skull are an example of fibrous joints.

Basic Joint Anatomy:

Understanding the anatomy of joints is crucial for comprehending how they function and how various conditions, such as arthritis or injuries, can impact joint health and mobility.

Articular Cartilage: Found at the ends of bones, this smooth, slippery tissue reduces friction and absorbs shock during movement.

Synovial Membrane: Lines the synovial cavity and secretes synovial fluid, which nourishes and lubricates the joint.

Joint Capsule: A tough, fibrous structure that encloses the joint, providing stability.

Ligaments: Tough bands of connective tissue that connect bones to each other, reinforcing the joint.

Joint Movement:

Joints allow for various types of movement, including flexion (bending), extension (straightening), abduction (moving away from the body's midline), adduction (moving toward the midline), and rotation.

Chapter 2

Understanding Arthritis

The Prevalence of Arthritis in Seniors

Arthritis is highly prevalent among seniors, posing a substantial health concern in aging populations. As individuals age, the risk of developing arthritis increases. According to the Centers for Disease Control and Prevention (CDC), approximately half of adults aged 65 years and older report being diagnosed with arthritis.

Osteoarthritis (OA), the most common form of arthritis, often develops with age as the protective cartilage on the ends of bones wears down over time. Rheumatoid arthritis (RA) and other inflammatory forms of arthritis also become more common in older age.

The impact of arthritis on seniors is profound, affecting their daily activities, mobility, and overall quality of life. Joint pain, stiffness, and limitations in movement can contribute to functional impairment and disability.

Efforts to address the prevalence of arthritis in seniors involve promoting awareness, early diagnosis, and implementing strategies for pain management and joint preservation. Lifestyle modifications, exercise programs, and medical interventions play a crucial role in mitigating the impact of arthritis and improving the well-being of seniors affected by this condition. As the global population continues to age, understanding and addressing arthritis in seniors become increasingly important for public health and healthcare systems.

The Journey to Finding Relief

The journey to finding relief from arthritis is often a multifaceted and personalized process, involving a combination of medical, lifestyle, and self-management strategies. Individuals experiencing arthritis navigate through several key steps on their path to relief:

1. **Diagnosis and Understanding:**

The journey typically begins with a thorough medical evaluation to determine the type and severity of arthritis. Understanding the specific form of arthritis is crucial for developing an effective treatment plan.

2. **Medical Interventions:**

Healthcare professionals may prescribe medications such as nonsteroidal anti-inflammatory drugs (NSAIDs), disease-modifying antirheumatic drugs (DMARDs), or biologics to manage symptoms and slow disease progression.

3. **Pain Management:**

Individuals often explore various pain management techniques, including over-the-counter or prescription pain relievers, topical treatments, and, in some cases, corticosteroid injections.

4. **Lifestyle Adjustments:**

Lifestyle modifications play a pivotal role. Regular exercise, tailored to individual abilities, helps maintain joint function and reduce stiffness. Weight management, a balanced diet, and adequate sleep contribute to overall well-being.

5. **Physical Therapy:**

Physical therapy is commonly recommended to improve joint flexibility, strengthen supporting muscles, and enhance overall mobility.

6. **Assistive Devices:**

Depending on the severity of arthritis, individuals may incorporate assistive devices such as braces, canes, or ergonomic tools to ease daily activities.

7. **Surgical Interventions:**

In advanced cases, surgical options like joint replacement may be considered to alleviate pain and improve joint function.

8. **Mind-Body Approaches:**

Mindfulness techniques, stress management, and complementary therapies like acupuncture or yoga can complement traditional treatments and enhance overall well-being.

9. **Regular Monitoring and Adaptation:**

Arthritis is a dynamic condition, and treatment plans may need adjustment over time. Regular check-ups with healthcare providers ensure that the approach remains effective and addresses evolving needs.

Boron in the Context of Holistic Health

Boron, often overlooked in the realm of nutrition, holds significant promise in contributing to holistic health. This essential trace mineral plays diverse roles in the body, impacting not only bone health but also various physiological processes. From cognitive function to joint health, Boron's influence extends across multiple systems, making it a valuable consideration in the pursuit of overall well-being within the framework of holistic health.

One of the key aspects of Boron's contribution to holistic health is its role in bone metabolism. By aiding in the absorption of calcium and magnesium, Boron supports bone density and strength. This becomes particularly relevant in the context of holistic health, where the interconnectedness of bodily systems is emphasized. Healthy bones contribute not only to physical mobility but also to a sense of vitality and independence, key components of a well-rounded approach to wellness.

In the realm of joint health, Boron's potential benefits for seniors, especially those grappling with arthritis, align with the holistic philosophy of addressing the root causes of health issues rather than merely managing symptoms. The Boron-rich recipes suggested earlier exemplify how incorporating this mineral into a balanced diet can be a flavorful and enjoyable part of a holistic health strategy.

Moreover, Boron's impact on cognitive function adds another layer to its holistic health implications. Research suggests that Boron may play a role in preserving cognitive function, an aspect crucial for maintaining mental well-being as individuals age. Integrating Boron into a holistic health plan acknowledges the importance of cognitive health alongside physical vitality.

In the context of holistic health, it's essential to consider the interconnectedness of nutritional choices, lifestyle, mental well-being, and the prevention of chronic conditions. Boron's multifaceted contributions align with this holistic approach, offering a potential avenue for individuals to address various facets of their health simultaneously.

As our understanding of nutrition and holistic health evolves, Boron emerges as a compelling element in the pursuit of overall well-being. From supporting bone health and joint function to potential cognitive benefits, Boron serves as a testament to the intricate connections within the body. While individual needs may vary, the incorporation of Boron into a holistic health strategy exemplifies a comprehensive approach to wellness that goes beyond isolated health concerns, embracing the concept of a healthy and vibrant life across all dimensions.

Chapter 3

Arthritis in the Golden Years

Current Approaches to Managing Arthritis in Seniors

The management of arthritis in seniors involves a combination of pharmacological and non-pharmacological approaches. Please note that new developments may have occurred since then, so it's always advisable to consult with healthcare professionals for the latest information. Here are some general approaches to managing arthritis in seniors:

1. **Medications:**

Pain Relievers (Analgesics): Acetaminophen is commonly used to manage pain, especially in osteoarthritis. Nonsteroidal anti-inflammatory drugs (NSAIDs) like ibuprofen and naproxen can help reduce inflammation and pain.

Disease-Modifying Antirheumatic Drugs (DMARDs): For rheumatoid arthritis, DMARDs such as methotrexate can slow down the progression of the disease and preserve joint function.

Biologics: In some cases, biologic drugs may be prescribed to target specific pathways involved in inflammation.

2. **Physical Therapy:**

Exercise Programs: Customized exercise programs can help improve joint function, reduce pain, and maintain flexibility. Low-impact exercises like swimming or walking are often recommended.

Joint Protection Techniques: Learning how to move and use joints in ways that reduce stress can help manage arthritis symptoms.

3. Occupational Therapy:

Adaptive Devices: Occupational therapists may recommend the use of assistive devices or tools to make daily tasks easier and reduce strain on joints.

4. Weight Management:

Maintaining a healthy weight is crucial for arthritis management, especially for weight-bearing joints. Weight loss can reduce the stress on joints and alleviate symptoms.

5. **Assistive Devices:**

Using canes, braces, or orthopedic shoes can help support joints and reduce strain during daily activities.

6. **Heat and Cold Therapy:**

Heat packs and cold compresses can be used to alleviate pain and inflammation. Hot showers or warm baths may also provide relief.

7. **Nutritional Support:**

A balanced diet with anti-inflammatory properties may help manage arthritis symptoms. Omega-3 fatty acids found in fish, flaxseed, and walnuts, for example, have anti-inflammatory effects.

8. **Joint Injections:**

In some cases, corticosteroid injections directly into affected joints can provide relief from inflammation and pain.

9. **Psychosocial Support:**

Dealing with chronic pain conditions can be mentally challenging. Support groups, counseling, or other forms of psychosocial support can be beneficial.

Medications and Their Side Effects

The medications used for arthritis management can have various side effects. It's crucial to note that the specific side effects can vary depending on the type of medication, the individual's health condition, and other factors.

Here's an overview of common medications used for arthritis and some of their potential side effects:

1. **Nonsteroidal Anti-Inflammatory Drugs (NSAIDs):**

Common examples: Ibuprofen, naproxen, diclofenac.

Side effects:

- Gastrointestinal issues: stomach pain, ulcers, bleeding.

- Cardiovascular issues: increased risk of heart attack or stroke.

- Kidney problems: reduced kidney function.

- Allergic reactions: rash, swelling, difficulty breathing.

2. **Acetaminophen:**

Side effects:

- Liver damage: especially with high doses or prolonged use.

3. **Disease-Modifying Antirheumatic Drugs (DMARDs):**

Common examples: Methotrexate, hydroxychloroquine, sulfasalazine.

Side effects:

- Liver problems: elevated liver enzymes.

- Bone marrow suppression: decreased blood cell counts.

- Increased risk of infection.

- Gastrointestinal issues.

4. **Biologic Response Modifiers (Biologics):**

Common examples: Etanercept, adalimumab, infliximab.

Side effects:

- Increased risk of infections.

- Allergic reactions: rash, itching, swelling.

- Injection site reactions.

- Liver problems.

5. **Corticosteroids:**

Common examples: Prednisone, cortisone.

Side effects:

- Bone loss: osteoporosis.

- Weight gain.

- Increased blood sugar levels: diabetes.

- Increased risk of infections.

- Mood changes: anxiety, depression.

6. **Analgesics (Pain Relievers):**

Common examples: Tramadol.

Side effects:

- Nausea, dizziness, constipation.

- Increased risk of seizures, especially at higher doses.

Physical Therapy and Exercise

Physical therapy and exercise are integral components of arthritis management, promoting joint flexibility, strength, and overall well-being.

Here's a more detailed look at how physical therapy and exercise contribute to arthritis management:

Physical Therapy:

1. Assessment and Individualized Plans:

Physical therapists assess the individual's specific condition, joint mobility, muscle strength, and functional abilities. They then create personalized treatment plans.

2. Range of Motion Exercises:

Specific exercises target maintaining or improving joint flexibility. This is crucial in preventing stiffness and enhancing the range of motion in affected joints.

3. **Strengthening Exercises:**

Targeted muscle strengthening helps support and stabilize joints affected by arthritis. Strengthening the muscles around the joints can reduce pain and improve overall function.

4. **Manual Therapy:**

Techniques such as massage and joint mobilization are used by physical therapists to alleviate pain, reduce muscle tension, and improve joint movement.

5. **Modalities for Pain Management:**

Physical therapists may use modalities such as heat, cold, ultrasound, or electrical stimulation to manage pain and inflammation.

6. **Posture and Body Mechanics:**

Education on proper posture and body mechanics is provided to minimize stress on joints during daily activities, reducing the risk of exacerbating arthritis symptoms.

7. **Balance and Coordination Training:**

Arthritis can impact balance and coordination. Physical therapists incorporate exercises to enhance these aspects, reducing the risk of falls and improving overall stability.

8. **Assistive Devices and Orthotics:**

Recommendations for the use of assistive devices or orthotics to support joints and improve mobility may be part of the therapy plan.

9. **Home Exercise Programs:**

Physical therapists often design home exercise programs to ensure continuity of care. Consistent practice of prescribed exercises is crucial for long-term benefits.

Exercise:

1. **Low-Impact Aerobic Exercise:**

Activities like walking, swimming, and cycling promote cardiovascular health without putting excessive stress on the joints. These exercises help maintain weight and reduce the risk of cardiovascular complications.

2. **Strength Training:**

Focused strength training exercises improve muscle tone and joint stability, reducing the impact of arthritis on daily activities.

3.   Flexibility and Stretching:

Regular stretching exercises enhance flexibility and reduce stiffness. This is particularly important in managing arthritis-related limitations in joint movement.

4. Joint-Friendly Activities:

Choosing activities that are gentle on the joints, such as water aerobics or Tai Chi, can provide the benefits of exercise without exacerbating arthritis symptoms.

5.   Weight Management:

Maintaining a healthy weight through regular exercise is crucial for individuals with arthritis, as excess weight can contribute to increased joint stress.

6. **Psychological Benefits:**

Exercise releases endorphins, which can positively impact mood and help manage stress, anxiety, and depression often associated with chronic conditions like arthritis.

Chapter 4

Boron - A Mineral of Interest

What Is Boron?

Boron is a chemical element with the symbol B and atomic number 5. It is a metalloid, meaning it has properties of both metals and nonmetals. Boron is found naturally in the environment, primarily in the form of borates, which are compounds that include boron, oxygen, and other elements.

Key points about boron include:

1.   **Occurrence:** Boron is relatively rare in the Earth's crust. It is often found in combination with other elements in minerals, the most common of which is borax.

2. **Uses:**

Industrial Applications: Boron compounds, especially borates, have various industrial applications. Boron is used in the production of glass, ceramics, and detergents.

Agriculture: Boron is an essential micronutrient for plants, and it is used in agriculture as boron fertilizers to improve crop yields.

Metallurgy: Boron is used in metallurgy to refine certain metals and alloys.

Nuclear Applications: Some boron compounds are used in nuclear reactors.

3. **Biological Importance:**

Boron is not considered an essential element for humans, but it may have potential health benefits. Some studies suggest that boron may play a role in bone health and metabolism.

4.   **Health Considerations:**

In trace amounts, boron is generally considered safe for humans. However, excessive intake can be toxic. Boron toxicity can cause symptoms such as nausea, vomiting, abdominal pain, and diarrhea.

Some people take boron supplements for purported health benefits, but it's essential to exercise caution and consult with a healthcare professional before taking any supplements.

5.   **Chemical Properties:**

Boron has interesting chemical properties. It does not occur freely in nature but is found in various borate minerals.

Boron compounds often exhibit unique structures and properties, making them useful in different applications.

6. **Isotopes:**

Boron has two stable isotopes: boron-10 and boron-11. Boron-10 is used in nuclear reactors for neutron capture, and boron-11 is the more abundant of the two stable isotopes.

7. **Flame Test:**

Boron compounds can impart a green color to a flame when burned, which can be used in a flame test for the presence of boron.

The History of Boron in Medicine

Here's an overview of the historical development of boron in medicine:

1.   **Early Observations:**

Boron's potential role in human health was not widely recognized until the late 20th century. Early observations noted that boron-rich areas seemed to have lower rates of certain health conditions.

2.   **Bone Health:**

Boron has been studied for its potential role in bone health. Some research suggests that boron may influence calcium and magnesium metabolism, which are essential for bone development.

3. **Arthritis and Joint Health:**

Boron has been investigated for its potential anti-inflammatory properties. Some studies have explored the use of boron supplements in managing inflammatory conditions such as arthritis. The idea is that boron may influence inflammatory pathways.

4. **Hormonal Regulation:**

Boron has been studied for its potential effects on hormones, particularly its interaction with estrogen. Some research has suggested that boron may play a role in hormone metabolism and may have implications for conditions such as osteoporosis.

5. **Brain Function:**

There is some research suggesting that boron may have a role in supporting cognitive function. However, the mechanisms behind this potential effect are not fully understood.

Antimicrobial Properties:

Boron compounds have been investigated for their antimicrobial properties. Some studies have explored the use of boron-containing compounds in the development of antimicrobial agents.

6. **Cancer Research:**

Boron compounds, particularly boron neutron capture therapy (BNCT), have been studied as a potential treatment for certain types of cancer. BNCT involves the use of boron-containing compounds that selectively accumulate in cancer cells and are then activated by neutron irradiation to destroy the tumor cells.

Chapter 5

Boron and Bone Health

Clinical Trials Involving Seniors

Clinical trials involving seniors are critical for advancing medical knowledge and developing effective interventions for age-related health conditions. Seniors, often defined as individuals aged 65 and older, are a diverse population with unique healthcare needs. Clinical trials involving seniors may focus on various aspects of health, including prevention, diagnosis, treatment, and quality of life.

Here are some common areas of research in clinical trials involving seniors:

1.   **Age-Related Diseases:**

Clinical trials may investigate treatments or interventions for age-related diseases such as osteoporosis, arthritis, cardiovascular diseases, Alzheimer's disease, and cancer.

2.   **Preventive Interventions:**

Trials may focus on preventive measures such as vaccines, lifestyle modifications, and medications to reduce the risk of certain diseases or conditions common in older adults.

3. **Medication Management:**

Studies may examine the safety, efficacy, and optimal dosage of medications commonly prescribed to seniors, considering factors such as metabolism changes and potential drug interactions.

4. **Cognitive Health:**

Clinical trials may assess interventions for maintaining cognitive function and preventing or treating conditions like dementia and Alzheimer's disease.

5. **Mobility and Physical Function:**

Research may target interventions to improve mobility, balance, and physical function in older adults, addressing issues related to falls and frailty.

6. **Palliative Care and End-of-Life Care:**

Trials may explore interventions to improve the quality of life for seniors with serious illnesses, including palliative care and end-of-life care strategies.

7. **Chronic Disease Management:**

Studies may investigate strategies for managing chronic conditions such as diabetes, hypertension, and chronic obstructive pulmonary disease (COPD) in older populations.

8. **Nutritional Interventions:**

Clinical trials may examine the impact of dietary interventions, nutritional supplements, or specific diets on health outcomes in seniors.

9. **Social and Mental Health:**

Research may focus on interventions to address social isolation, depression, and mental health issues prevalent among seniors.

10. **Technology and Aging:**

Trials may explore the use of technology, such as telemedicine, wearable devices, and smart home technologies, to enhance healthcare delivery and improve seniors' quality of life.

The Impact of Boron on Calcium and Magnesium Metabolism

Boron has been studied for its potential impact on calcium and magnesium metabolism, particularly in relation to bone health. While the mechanisms are not fully understood, research suggests that boron may play a role in the absorption and utilization of calcium and magnesium in the body.

Here are some key points related to the impact of boron on calcium and magnesium metabolism:

1.   **Calcium Metabolism:**

Boron may influence calcium metabolism by enhancing the absorption and utilization of calcium in the bones. Research has suggested that boron supplementation may positively affect bone mineral density.

2.   **Bone Health:**

Boron is believed to play a role in bone health, and it may interact with calcium and magnesium in bone metabolism. Some studies have explored the effects of boron on bone density and strength.

3.   **Magnesium Metabolism:**

Boron is thought to enhance magnesium absorption and retention. Magnesium is a crucial mineral for various physiological functions, including bone health, muscle function, and nerve transmission.

4.   **Hormonal Regulation:**

Boron may influence hormonal regulation, including the activity of hormones such as estrogen and vitamin D, which are involved in calcium and magnesium metabolism.

5. **Research Findings:**

Studies, such as those conducted by Hunt et al. and Nielsen et al., have explored the effects of boron deprivation and supplementation on calcium and magnesium metabolism. These studies suggested that boron deprivation could adversely affect bone health and mineral metabolism, while boron supplementation might have positive effects.

6. **Potential Benefits for Osteoporosis:**

Osteoporosis, a condition characterized by decreased bone density and increased risk of fractures, has been a focus of research related to boron. Some studies propose that boron supplementation might have potential benefits for individuals at risk of osteoporosis.

7. **Synergistic Effects:**

Boron's interactions with calcium and magnesium are likely complex and involve multiple mechanisms. Boron may act synergistically with these minerals to support bone health and overall metabolic processes.

8. **Dietary Sources:**

Boron is naturally present in certain foods, including fruits, vegetables, nuts, and legumes. Consuming a balanced diet with these foods contributes to overall mineral intake, including boron.

Boron and Arthritis: What the Research Says

Research on boron and arthritis suggests potential benefits. Some studies propose that boron may have anti-inflammatory properties and could contribute to symptom relief and improved joint function in arthritis patients. However, more research is needed to establish specific mechanisms and optimal dosages for effective arthritis management. Always consult with healthcare professionals before considering boron supplementation for arthritis.

Chapter 6

Foods High in Boron

Boron is found in varying amounts in a variety of foods. While it's not classified as an essential nutrient, some studies suggest that adequate boron intake may have potential health benefits.

Here is a list of foods that are relatively high in boron:

1. **Fruits:**

   - Apples
   - Grapes
   - Oranges
   - Avocado
   - Prunes
   - Bananas

- Pears

2. Vegetables:

- Broccoli

- Carrots

- Cauliflower

- Spinach

- Kale

- Onions

- Potatoes

3. Nuts and Seeds:

- Almonds

- Peanuts

- Hazelnuts

- Sunflower seeds

- Pumpkin seeds

- Walnuts

4. Legumes:

- Soybeans

- Lentils

- Chickpeas

- Peas

5. Whole Grains:

- Brown rice

- Quinoa

- Barley

- Whole wheat

6. Dried Fruits:

- Raisins

- Apricots

7. **Beverages:**

    - Red wine

    - Coffee

8. **Herbs and Spices:**

    - Thyme

    - Turmeric

    - Cumin

9. **Dairy and Dairy Alternatives:**

    - Milk

    - Cheese

    - Yogurt

    - Plant-based milk alternatives fortified with boron

10. **Meat:**

- Fish

- Chicken

- Beef

- Turkey

Chapter 7

14days Boron-Friendly Meal Plan

Week 1

Day 1:

- **Breakfast:** Greek yogurt with walnuts and honey, whole-grain toast.

- **Lunch:** Quinoa salad with spinach, cherry tomatoes, cucumber, and feta cheese.

- **Dinner:** Baked salmon with lemon and herbs, steamed broccoli, and sweet potatoes.

Day 2:

- **Breakfast:** Oatmeal with sliced bananas and almonds.

- **Lunch:** Lentil soup with whole-grain crackers.

- **Dinner:** Grilled chicken breast, brown rice, mixed vegetables.

Day 3:

- **Breakfast:** Smoothie with kale, pineapple, Greek yogurt, and chia seeds.

- **Lunch:** Chickpea and vegetable stir-fry with quinoa.

- **Dinner:** Baked cod with a side of roasted Brussels sprouts and quinoa.

Day 4:

- **Breakfast:** Whole-grain toast with avocado and poached eggs.

- **Lunch:** Spinach and strawberry salad with grilled chicken.

- **Dinner:** Turkey meatballs with tomato sauce, whole-grain pasta, and a side of green beans.

Day 5:

- **Breakfast:** Cottage cheese with sliced peaches and a sprinkle of sunflower seeds.

- **Lunch:** Brown rice bowl with black beans, corn, avocado, and salsa.

- **Dinner:** Baked sweet and sour tofu with broccoli and quinoa.

Day 6:

- **Breakfast:** Whole-grain waffles with fresh berries and a dollop of Greek yogurt.

- **Lunch:** Quinoa and vegetable stuffed peppers.

- **Dinner:** Grilled shrimp with a side of asparagus and wild rice.

Day 7:

- **Breakfast:** Smoothie bowl with mixed berries, banana, and granola.

- **Lunch:** Turkey and vegetable wrap with a side of carrot sticks.

- **Dinner:** Baked chicken thighs with lemon and herbs, roasted sweet potatoes, and green beans.

Week 2

Day 8:

- **Breakfast:** Scrambled eggs with sautéed spinach and whole-grain toast.

- **Lunch:** Quinoa and black bean bowl with diced tomatoes, avocado, and a lime dressing.

- **Dinner:** Baked trout with lemon and dill, sweet potato wedges, and steamed broccoli.

Day 9:

- **Breakfast:** Whole-grain pancakes with blueberries and a dollop of Greek yogurt.

- **Lunch:** Lentil and vegetable curry with brown rice.

- **Dinner:** Grilled vegetable skewers with chicken, quinoa, and a side of mixed greens.

Day 10:

- **Breakfast:** Overnight oats with sliced strawberries, chia seeds, and a drizzle of honey.

- **Lunch:** Chickpea and quinoa salad with cherry tomatoes, cucumber, and feta cheese.

- **Dinner:** Baked cod with a herb crust, roasted Brussels sprouts, and wild rice.

Day 11:

- **Breakfast:** Whole-grain bagel with smoked salmon, cream cheese, and capers.

- **Lunch:** Spinach and feta stuffed chicken breast, quinoa, and a side of roasted sweet potatoes.

- **Dinner:** Shrimp stir-fry with broccoli, snap peas, and brown rice.

Day 12:

- **Breakfast:** Greek yogurt parfait with granola, mixed berries, and a sprinkle of almonds.

- **Lunch:** Turkey and vegetable kebabs with quinoa and a Greek salad.

- **Dinner:** Baked chicken thighs with rosemary, sweet potato mash, and steamed green beans.

Day 13:

- **Breakfast:** Whole-grain toast with avocado, cherry tomatoes, and a poached egg.

- **Lunch:** Quinoa and black bean stuffed bell peppers.

- **Dinner:** Grilled salmon with a honey-mustard glaze, roasted Brussels sprouts, and quinoa.

Day 14:

- **Breakfast:** Smoothie with kale, pineapple, Greek yogurt, and a handful of walnuts.

- **Lunch:** Lentil and vegetable soup with a side of whole-grain crackers.

- **Dinner:** Baked tofu with teriyaki glaze, brown rice, and stir-fried vegetables.

Chapter 8

Boron-Rich Recipes for Seniors

These recipes are designed to be nutritious and incorporate ingredients rich in boron. Adjust portion sizes and ingredients based on individual dietary needs and preferences.

Boron-Boosted Avocado Salad:

Ingredients:

- Avocado

- Spinach

- Cherry tomatoes

- Sunflower seeds

Instructions:

- Toss spinach, sliced avocado, halved cherry tomatoes, and sunflower seeds in a bowl.

- Dress with a light vinaigrette.

Quinoa and Broccoli Stir-Fry:

Ingredients:

- Quinoa

- Broccoli florets

- Carrots

- Soy sauce

Instructions:

- Cook quinoa according to package instructions.

  - Stir-fry broccoli and carrots in a pan, add cooked quinoa, and drizzle with soy sauce.

Boron-Infused Lentil Soup:

Ingredients:

  - Lentils

  - Spinach

  - Carrots

  - Tomatoes

Instructions:

  - Cook lentils with diced tomatoes, carrots, and spinach.

  - Season with herbs and spices for flavor.

Sweet Potato and Kale Casserole:

Ingredients:

- Sweet potatoes

- Kale

- Onion

- Garlic

Instructions:

- Layer sliced sweet potatoes, sautéed kale, onions, and garlic in a baking dish.

- Bake until sweet potatoes are tender.

Boron-Enriched Salmon Patties:

Ingredients:

- Canned salmon

- Eggs

- Almond flour

- Dill

Instructions:

- Mix canned salmon, beaten eggs, almond flour, and dill.

- Form into patties and cook until golden.

Cauliflower and Walnut Salad:

Ingredients:

- Cauliflower

- Walnuts

- Cranberries

- Feta cheese

Instructions:

- Roast cauliflower, mix with chopped walnuts, cranberries, and crumbled feta.

Boron-Boosted Berry Smoothie:

Ingredients:

- Mixed berries

- Almond milk

- Chia seeds

- Greek yogurt

Instructions:

- Blend berries, almond milk, chia seeds, and Greek yogurt until smooth.

Baked Cod with Lemon and Asparagus:

Ingredients:

- Cod fillets

- Asparagus

- Lemon

- Olive oil

Instructions:

- Place cod and asparagus on a baking sheet, drizzle with olive oil and lemon juice, bake until fish flakes easily.

Spinach and Mushroom Omelette:

Ingredients:

- Eggs

- Spinach

- Mushrooms

- Cheese

Instructions:

- Sauté spinach and mushrooms, pour beaten eggs over, cook until set, sprinkle with cheese.

Boron-Rich Banana Walnut Muffins: -

Ingredients:

- Bananas –
- Whole wheat flour –
- Walnuts –
- Greek yogurt –

Instructions:

- Mash bananas,

- mix with whole wheat flour, chopped walnuts, and Greek yogurt.
- Bake in muffin cups until golden.

Quinoa and Black Bean Stuffed Peppers:

Ingredients:

- Bell peppers
- Quinoa
- Black beans
- Corn

Instructions:

Cook quinoa and mix with black beans and corn. Stuff into halved bell peppers and bake until peppers are tender.

Boron-Boosted Greek Salad:

Ingredients:

- Cucumber

- Feta cheese

- Kalamata olives

- Red onion

Instructions:

- Combine diced cucumber,
  crumbled feta, sliced olives,
  and red onion. Drizzle with
  olive oil.

Lentil and Vegetable Curry:

- Ingredients:

- Red lentils

- Mixed vegetables (bell peppers, carrots, peas)

- Coconut milk

- Curry spices

Instructions:

- Cook lentils and vegetables in coconut milk, season with curry spices.

Baked Sweet Potato Fries:

Ingredients:

- Sweet potatoes

- Olive oil

- Rosemary

- Sea salt

Instructions:

- Cut sweet potatoes into fries,
  toss with olive oil, rosemary,
  and sea salt. Bake until crispy.

Boron-Infused Berry Parfait:

- Ingredients:

  - Mixed berries

  - Greek yogurt

  - Granola

  - Honey

- Instructions:

  - Layer Greek yogurt with mixed
    berries and granola. Drizzle
    with honey.

Broccoli and Cheddar Quiche:

Ingredients:

- Broccoli

- Cheddar cheese

- Eggs

- Pie crust

Instructions:

- Steam broccoli, mix with shredded cheddar, pour into a pie crust with beaten eggs, and bake.

Mediterranean Chickpea Salad:

Ingredients:

- Chickpeas

- Cherry tomatoes

- Cucumber

- Red onion

Instructions:

- Combine chickpeas, halved cherry tomatoes, diced cucumber, and red onion. Dress with olive oil and lemon.

Almond-Crusted Chicken Tenders:

Ingredients:

- Chicken tenders

- Almond flour

- Egg

- Garlic powder

Instructions:

- Dip chicken tenders in beaten egg, coat with a mixture of almond flour and garlic powder, bake until golden.

Boron-Rich Berry Smoothie Bowl:

Ingredients:

- Mixed berries

- Spinach

- Almond milk

- Chia seeds

Instructions:

- Blend berries, spinach, almond milk, and chia seeds. Pour into a bowl, top with granola.

Quinoa and Kale Stuffed Acorn Squash:

Ingredients:

- Acorn squash

- Quinoa

- Kale

- Pecans

Instructions:

- Roast acorn squash, fill with a mixture of quinoa, sautéed kale, and chopped pecans.

Boron-Infused Brussels Sprouts Salad:

Ingredients:

- Brussels sprouts

- Cranberries

- Pecans

- Feta cheese

Instructions:

- Shred Brussels sprouts and toss with cranberries, chopped pecans, and crumbled feta. Drizzle with balsamic vinaigrette.

Lemon-Garlic Shrimp and Asparagus Stir-Fry:

Ingredients:

- Shrimp

- Asparagus

- Garlic

- Lemon

Instructions:

- Stir-fry shrimp and asparagus with minced garlic, squeeze lemon over the top. Serve over brown rice.

Boron-Rich Berry Chia Pudding:

Ingredients:

- Mixed berries

- Chia seeds

- Almond milk

- Honey

Instructions:

- Mix chia seeds with almond milk, refrigerate until pudding-like. Top with mixed berries and a drizzle of honey.

Spinach and Mushroom Whole Wheat Pasta:

Ingredients:

- Whole wheat pasta

- Spinach

- Mushrooms

- Parmesan cheese

Instructions:

- Cook whole wheat pasta, sauté spinach and mushrooms, toss together. Sprinkle with Parmesan.

Boron-Boosted Oatmeal with Almonds and Dried Apricots:

Ingredients:

- Oats

- Almonds

- Dried apricots

- Cinnamon

Instructions:

- Cook oats, top with sliced
  almonds, chopped dried
  apricots, and a sprinkle of
  cinnamon.

Mediterranean Stuffed Bell Peppers:

Ingredients:

- Bell peppers

- Ground turkey

- Quinoa

- Tomatoes

Instructions:

- Cook quinoa and brown ground turkey. Mix with diced tomatoes, stuff into bell peppers, and bake.

Boron-Infused Spinach and Feta Frittata:

Ingredients:

- Eggs

- Spinach

- Feta cheese

- Red bell pepper

Instructions:

- Whisk eggs, mix with sautéed spinach, crumbled feta, and diced red bell pepper. Bake until set.

94

Cauliflower and Broccoli Gratin:

Ingredients:

- Cauliflower

- Broccoli

- Gruyere cheese

- Milk

Instructions:

- Steam cauliflower and broccoli, layer in a baking dish with a mixture of milk and grated Gruyere. Bake until bubbly.

Boron-Rich Pistachio Crusted Chicken:

Ingredients:

- Chicken breasts

- Pistachios

- Dijon mustard

- Lemon

Instructions:

- Coat chicken breasts in a mixture of crushed pistachios, Dijon mustard, and lemon zest. Bake until cooked through.

Avocado and Pomegranate Quinoa Salad:

- Ingredients:

    - Quinoa

    - Avocado

    - Pomegranate seeds

    - Mint

Instructions:

- Cook quinoa, toss with diced avocado, pomegranate seeds, and chopped mint. Drizzle with olive oil.

Chapter 9

Conclusion

In conclusion, the potential benefits of Boron as a complementary element in the management of arthritis among seniors present a promising avenue for enhanced well-being and improved quality of life. As we've explored, Boron is believed to play a crucial role in bone health and joint function, two areas profoundly impacted by arthritis. The various Boron-rich recipes provided earlier not only offer a flavorful and diverse range of meals for seniors but also strategically incorporate ingredients that contribute to increased Boron intake.

The synergy between Boron and other essential nutrients found in these recipes may provide seniors with arthritis an opportunity to address joint discomfort and promote overall joint health. While it's essential to underscore the importance of consulting healthcare professionals for personalized advice, these Boron-rich recipes offer a delicious and accessible means for seniors to integrate this element into their diets.

Moreover, the potential economic aspect of Boron as a supplement or a dietary consideration in arthritis management should not be overlooked. Given the growing market for health-conscious and age-specific nutritional solutions, there exists a unique opportunity for entrepreneurs and healthcare providers to explore the development of Boron-enriched dietary supplements or specialized meal plans tailored to seniors with arthritis.

As we continue to advance our understanding of nutritional science and its implications for aging populations, the incorporation of Boron into arthritis management strategies may not only prove beneficial for seniors but also present a lucrative prospect for businesses in the health and wellness sector. In the pursuit of a holistic approach to senior health, Boron stands out as a potentially valuable and profitable component in the ongoing dialogue surrounding arthritis care.

www.ingramcontent.com/pod-product-compliance
Lightning Source LLC
Chambersburg PA
CBHW070837260726
48660CB00005B/2067